101

Ways

To

Get

Fat

BY

Mrs. MANJU SETHIYA

[ZHINGOORA BOOKS]

Mrs. MANJU SETHIYA

After waking up, take heavy breakfast.

1. In afternoon, take heavy brunch.

2. In night take heavy dinner.

3. Use fried stuff in your meal.

Mrs. MANJU SETHIYA

4. Always drink creamy milk, don't drink skimmed one.

5. Use potatoes in your diet. Its good store of carbohydrates and rich in starch.

6. Try to be always happy.

Mrs. MANJU SETHIYA

7.   Take complete sleep of 8 hours.

8.   Eat whenever you feel hungry.

9.   Sleep after eating food to digest it properly. So, whenever you are awake you can eat more.

Mrs. MANJU SETHIYA

10. Don't take any tension or stress.

11. Always remain miles away from dieting.

12. Use fatty oils in your meals.

13. Eat at irregular times.

Mrs. MANJU SETHIYA

14. Use cream, cheese, paneer, and butter in your diet.

15. Get rid of your stress or tension by sharing with someone you find suitable.

16. Eat fast foods. As they are tasty and

you like to eat again and again.

17. Drink milk by adding Ghee.

18. Don't remove starch from rice and potatoes.

19. Take B12 tablets (Please consult your

doctor before any
medication)

20. Eat wholegrain
wheat.

21. Drink milk with
bournvita.

22. Take two
bananas daily with
milk.

23. Take tonic which increase your appetite.

24. Do jogging, exercise and yoga.

25. Drink milk and eggs everyday.

26. Use groundnut and peanut butter in your food.

Mrs. MANJU SETHIYA

27. Take desserts
after meal.

28. Take pulses in
your diet.

29. Eat sugar made
stuffs.

30. Eat potatoes
daily.

31. Eat food stuffs
rich in calories.

Mrs. MANJU SETHIYA

32. Take fruits after meal. As, it is good for digestion.

33. Eat pizza, burger and sandwiches.

34. Eat pancakes and biscuits.

35. Take fish in your diet.

36. Choose many items as much as possible while taking your Dinner.

37. Make obese people friends. So you don't feel isolated.

38. Keep your teeth healthy.

Mrs. MANJU SETHIYA

39. Keep your behavior jolly and joyful.

40. Keep proper medication to increase your diet.

41. Keep away yourself from people who quarrel and incite you.

Mrs. MANJU SETHIYA

42. Read jokes.

43. Read health magazines.

44. Make your dishes in fatty oils.

45. Eat different cuisines.

46. Always be with people who love eating.

Mrs. MANJU SETHIYA

47. Do things which make you happy.

48. Eat up to last bit of space left in your stomach.

49. Read article on health progress.

50. Drink alcohol.

51. Eat dry fruits.

52. Drink cold drinks.

53. Take bread and butter.

54. Take Aaloo Paratha. [Bread filled with stuffed potatoes, widely used in India]

55. Eat more than you feel.

56. Eat snacks while watching TV, movie and reading.

57. Do not avoid food while you are hungry.

58. Don't do fasting.

59. Try different types of cheese.

60. Do sitting work.

Mrs. MANJU SETHIYA

61. Make your meal tasty.

62. Use spices in your food to increase your diet.

63. Use Ghee. It is good source of fat.

64. Take curd rice.

65. Use soybean's products in your meal.

66. Use rice in your diet. As it will quickly digest.

67. Eat cheese sandwich.

68. Watch TV while eating.

Mrs. MANJU SETHIYA

69. Eat favourite dishes.

70. Use vehicle trip rather than walking.

71. Don't take stress. As it will cause depression.

72. Always keep food items with you. So, you can eat

whenever you are feeling hungry.

73. Eat cake and pastries.

74. Eat snacks regularly.

75. Eat fried cashew nuts.

76. Eat halwa.

77. Eat food items which have starch.

78. Try new restaurant every week. It will create excitement about food.

79. Attend party and give party.

80. Don't be with misers, which afraid to do expense.

81. Take cooking classes to learn new dishes.

82. Always do discussion on food stuffs.

83. Watch cook shows.

84. Set timer to inform you about schedule of food stuffs.

85. Make food menu for your week ahead.

86. Try to mingle with the people of other religion. As they have new cuisines to offer you.

87. Try to compensate the calorie loss after exercise.

Mrs. MANJU SETHIYA

88. Take long walk
after your meal.
89. Try to do more
and more body
work. So that your
body will absorbs
the food you have
consumed.

Mrs. MANJU SETHIYA

90. Try to be away from thin people than yourself

91. Enjoy the food while eating.

92. Try to laugh one hour in a day.

93. Add cream/butter in the soup.

Mrs. MANJU SETHIYA

94. Try to eat Indian curries as they are rich in calories.

95. Drink more carbonated drink because they contain high calories.

96. Drink Coffee.

Mrs. MANJU SETHIYA

97. Eat dairy products.

98. Try sitting around whole day.

99. Go to every event that serves food.

100. Read this book daily.

Mrs. MANJU SETHIYA

101 Ways To Get Fat

Mrs. MANJU SETHIYA

End of the Book

Mrs. MANJU SETHIYA

www.ingramcontent.com/pod-product-compliance
Lightning Source LLC
Chambersburg PA
CBHW060020300526
45794CB00003B/1231